My Anti-Inflammatory Diet Cookbook

Heal Your Body With 82 Delicious Recipes

Written by

Donna Barrow

Table Of Contents

Introduction

Heal Inflammation with Anti-Inflammatory Diet

Benefits of an Anti-Inflammatory Diet

The anti-inflammatory diet is good for weight loss too. You might lose weight while on the diet. It is a new way of eating that has all the nutrients and minerals and proteins you need to be healthy.

It will give you a fresh perspective on your life, even if it only lasts three weeks.

The anti-inflammatory diet will help you feel better. It will have nutrients that fight inflammation and help you heal.

You will start to look and feel better. Your skin will have a nice glow, and your body will work how it should.

If you follow the anti-inflammatory diet, you will get all these benefits.

But first you need to understand yourself so that you know what foods are best for your body and why.

The main signs of inflammation are: warmth, redness, pain, swelling and loss of muscle function.

These symptoms depend on the part of your body that is inflamed and what caused it.

Some of the signs of chronic inflammation are:

- Gastrointestinal problems like diarrhea, constipation, and acid reflux disease
- Body pain
- Fatigue
- Insomnia
- Weight gain
- Frequent infections
- Mood disorders like anxiety and depression.

If you have inflammation, you might have symptoms like a rash or tiredness. Inflammation can be caused by different problems in the body.

If you have arthritis, it causes pain in the joints. The symptoms are sometimes tingling, pain, stiffness and swelling.

Inflammatory bowel disease usually affects the digestive system. If someone has it, they might have bleeding ulcers, anemia, weight loss, bloating, pains or stomach aches.

Multiple sclerosis also affects the myelin sheath of nerve cells. It includes problems when passing out stool and blurred eyesight.

If you have any of these symptoms, it may be inflammation. It maybe is related to joints like arthritis. You can know if it's arthritis if you have swelling and pain in the joint.
There are other problems that cause soreness too, but there is not always a problem with them. For example, acute inflammation is important for recovery from an injury like a twisted ankle and swollen knee or back.

It is easy to find out if someone has chronic inflammation. There are signs and causes of it that people can see. Insomnia, traits in your genes, food intake, and other individual habits can cause it. Inflammation resulting from allergies also may happen in your gut.

Below are some of the possibilities that you may be having it:

- If you always feel tired, and it doesn't seem to make a difference whether or not you sleep well at night
- Sometimes you might feel pain in your joints. That could be because you have arthritis
- Do you have pain in your gut? The pain may cause inflammation. The inflammation might make you cramp and have a lot of gas
- If there's an infection in your body, you might have swollen lymph nodes. These are found under your neck, near your armpits, and near your groin. They swell up if there is something wrong with your body and the defense system has noticed it. The nodes become smaller when the infection goes away and you heal

- Do you have a stuffy nose? If so, it might be because you have a toothache in your nose
- Sometimes, the surface of your skin may be sore because of inflammation.

Inflammation caused by pathogens, bacteria, viruses, or any other external influence is a corrective measure used by the human body when it has incurred an injury.

The protective measure helps you to heal. You can have immune cells, blood vessels, and white blood cells to help the aggravated body part fix the damaged cell. Then you can heal. However, in some cases, our immune system causes inflammation even when there are no external things to fight (For example, arthritis).

This means that the body will treat the disease like it is regular tissue disintegration. This can cause pain and inflammation.
Inflammation can be dealt with in many ways. One of the most common is to add food items with anti-inflammatory benefits to your diet.

Research has shown that diet food that helps with inflammation is more effective than medicines.

People who live a healthy lifestyle with regular exercise and eat an anti-inflammatory diet are not only healthier but often live longer. This is true for people of all kinds, but also for athletes who often get injured easily.

Here is a guide for inflammation. It is about how it affects your body and what you need to know. This book is about making the process of starting an anti-inflammatory diet more spontaneous. You will find a lot of recipes in it too.

With all the information on the internet and in books, it can be hard to know what is true. That makes things difficult when you are already feeling pain.

This book will help you to understand inflammation, it is written in a way that is easy to understand. The author of this book is not trying to show that he is smart. He wants to teach you through simple language.

The recipes mentioned in this book are easy to follow. You can easily get ingredients that have anti-inflammation properties from the store.

By the time you are ready to eat, you will have learned a lot about how to help your inflammation.

The book clears away myths and offers a no-nonsense approach to inflammation. This helps you get rid of the pain that's been bothering you for a long time.

Inflammation is the body's natural response to protect itself.

Inflammation is something your body does to fight back against a disease or an injury. Inflammation can happen to all people. Sometimes, it is noticeable outside of the body but other times it's not.

When the body has certain conditions, inflammation can happen. Inflammation is a way that our body tells us to be safe. If it weren't for inflammation, lots of people would stay hurt for a long time or not heal at all.

Inflammation happens when we come into contact with something that our body does not like. This can include an attack by a pathogen, or injured cells due to injury. It may also be caused by something irritating, such as a chemical or other agent.

Inflammation in our bodies is carried out by the cells that are part of our immune system, as well as blood vessels. These cells and blood vessels all work together to make inflammation happen.

Inflammation is the first defense in your body. It prevents the pathogen from causing more harm to your body. Inflammation also helps with clearing away dead cells around the spot where you were hurt. Inflammation makes the body heal faster. Some signs of inflammation are heat, swelling, redness, and pain.

There are two types of inflammation: acute and chronic. Acute inflammation is what occurs in a break from skin, because it can help your immune system better attack the bacteria entering through open wound. In contrast, chronic may be due to an underlying health problem like cancer or metabolic syndrome.

Acute inflammation is a condition that happens when someone gets an outside attack. The body responds by making more plasma and leukocyte cells. During this process, a special kind of white blood cell, called granulocytes, is flown into the injured tissues. This helps to calm the area. This process can also be called an inflammatory response.

Acute inflammation is the first thing your body does when you get hurt. It is short and it only lasts for a few days before the injury heals. Cytokines and chemokines help neutrophils and macrophages to go to the injured area so that it can heal. If there are six weeks of inflammation, then that is called acute inflammation.

When you have pain and inflammation, it is best to get it treated. Acute inflammation lasts for a few days or weeks. But chronic inflammation can last for months or years. In the case of chronic inflammation, the body gets worse and different cells (macrophages, plasma cells and lymphocytes) replace neutrophils. Some common cases of chronic inflammation are diabetes, cardiovascular ailments, allergies, and pulmonary disease. Problems with chronic inflammation might be because of obesity, unhealthy eating habits or smoking. Stress is also a problem.

Inflammation is an injury that often happens to athletes and people who exercise. This usually happens when the body is in pain.

Your body can heal from inflammation. But when the pain and inflammation lasts for a long time, look into what you're eating and doing. You might not eat things that will make your inflammation worse or do things that will make it better.

Inflammation can happen in the body when there are irritants or other things that the body cannot easily process. If there is inflammation, it might not be treated on time and then it could lead to a chronic disorder.

Some foods, like processed sugar, refined carbs, alcohol, and processed meat or fat can make inflammation worse.

Inflammation is something that we all face. It can happen to people who are very active, like athletes and health enthusiasts.

Inflammation is something that happens when the body gets hurt. It means the skin will get red and swollen, and it can be painful. You should not ignore it because it might be a sign of something serious going on inside your body.

Therefore, the inflammation can be caused by both an outer blow and an inner attack. This means that your body cannot heal properly.

There are many things that cause inflammation. Some of them are:

Chemical injury: If the body is exposed to harsh chemicals, it can lead to redness and swelling in the skin.

Pathogens: These are organisms that can cause a disease. The human body already has microbes that can make the immune system not work as well. If not treated for a long time, the microbes start to fight and make the immune system weaker. But if you get these organisms from outside your body, they will cause problems with your immune system right away.

External injuries: When the body suffers an injury from the outside, it might result in a wound. If the wound is not cared for or if you don't treat it on time, it may lead to inflammation and redness. A scrape of any kind on any part of your body will lead to these kinds of wounds that can cause inflammation.

Medical conditions: If you don't get treatment for a disease, then the inflammation can get worse. Different diseases make different parts of your body hurt. For example, cystitis makes your bladder hurt, bronchitis makes your lungs hurt, otitis media makes your ears hurt and dermatitis makes the skin around it burn and itch.

Diseases can make it hard to identify the injury that caused it. But there are some common traits that you might find in injured people.

Some symptoms of inflammation that happen to a person are:

Redness: The most common symptom of inflammation is when your body turns red. When an outside agent, such as a bug, touchs your skin and makes it turn red. Doctors might need special equipment if the injury is inside your body.

Pain: In some cases, inflammation can also lead to extreme pain in the human body or an irritated area. The level of pain indicates how serious the blow or injury is. This pain may be from outside impacts, but it might happen inside your body too. If you feel this type of pain, do not treat it lightly and go see a doctor if it doesn't go away on its own.

Loss of function: In some cases, chronic injuries can cause people to lose their ability to do things. For example, people may have pain or inflammation in their joints. They might not be able to move because of the pain. Another example is when they have a hard time breathing because of inflammation in their lungs.

Swelling: This is a symptom of inflammation. When the body's immune system starts to heal an injury, it causes swelling in a particular place.

Heat: If your body part is hurt or gets an infection, sometimes the body will feel hot. Sometimes the body also develops a fever and raises the temperature. This is another sign of inflammation.
Flu-like symptoms can be a sign of inflammation too. Some common signs are fever, chills, cough, shortness of breath, cold and fatigue.

Inflammation does not always cause the symptoms mentioned. On occasion, inflammation can be an internal problem, and is not known by the person.

Doctors should be consulted if the person is not feeling well. Some inflammations do not have any symptoms until they are diagnosed by a professional.

Inflammation can make it hard for your body to fight off diseases. It can also make you more tired and it might cause some pain.

Inflammation is a problem that many people have. If it does not go away in a few days and you do not get treatment, it can make other problems happen in your body.

Inflammation is when your immune system is busy. This happens because you might have hurt yourself, for example. Your immune system works to heal the area quickly. The area becomes red and white blood cells come to help fix it.

The body does the same thing for an injury inside the body. It is good to take these steps, but if the inflammation is not going away or it is taking a long time to go away, then there might be an illness in your body that prevents your body from fighting back on its own. This could happen because you might not have enough white blood cells or because you didn't get enough sleep.

In some cases, it can take longer for injury to heal because the person has a big injury and inflammation is harder to heal. They should go talk to someone who knows about this and not let the problem get worse.

Inflammation sometimes does not work the way it should. The immune response to inflammation can happen even if the body did not suffer any injury.

Therefore, the body of a person gets inflammation. This will not get better because the immune system cannot heal it for long. This causes pain and other disorders in the human body.

Some people can get inflammation from obesity, stress, or other autoimmune disorders. This kind of abnormal inflammation is identified as chronic inflammation.

When left unattended, inflammation can lead to a lot of health problems. Some of the most common are heart ailments, arthritis, depression, cancer and Alzheimer's disease.

Acute inflammation has been shown to go away in a short time, but chronic inflammation can lead to many disorders and affect the healthy living of a person. Over time, chronic inflammation can also cause the reverse immune system response.

The immune system protects your body and keeps it healthy. Sometimes, the immune system can start to attack your own body.

Diabetes, cancer, and rheumatoid arthritis are some of the most common diseases that cause unlawful inflammation.

If you have an inflammation, you should talk to a doctor. The doctor will help with medicine and other things so the problem does not spread and disturb your immunity.

One of the best ways to fight inflammation is to exercise and eat healthy. This way, you avoid things that cause or make it worse. You should avoid foods like ice cream or fried food because they can cause or aggravate inflammation.

Avoid red meat, processed carbs, deep-fried foods, and sugar. Instead eat vegetables, fruit that is in season, nuts and fish.

Doing things like exercising and sleeping well will help you to stay calm. It is also important to not let your mind get stressed.

Let's Create an Effective Anti-Inflammatory Diet

Guidelines for the Anti-Inflammatory Diet

It has been proven that to fight inflammation, a person should focus more on their kitchen and healthy food than go to the doctor's. Doctors are important if someone develops chronic inflammation. But no one can counter the benefits of eating healthy food, which is what doctors also recommend.

An anti-inflammatory diet is not very specific. It replaces all food items with processed carbs, deep-fried foods, red meat, alcohol and processed sugar and replaces them with fruits and green leafy vegetables, fatty, omega-3 fatty acids, whole grains, lean protein and some spices.

There are no certain guidelines for what type of diet to do. But there are some foods that may make inflammation worse, like sugar or gluten.

Dairy products, processed foods, foods with added sugar or salt, unhealthy oils, processed carbs, baked goods, processed snacks, legumes, eggs, premade desserts, red meat like steaks and processed meat, alcohol including wine and carbonated sugar beverage too are not good for people who have inflammation because they will make it worse.

A person who has decided to go on an anti-inflammatory diet should eat all natural food, like vegetables and fruits. They need to eat a well-balanced meal that includes foods with antioxidants, like berries and beans. And they should not eat things that are rich in acids, like sugar.

Some research has shown that people can have a more anti-inflammatory diet by carefully selecting between the Mediterranean diet and the DASH diet. They should include fresh fruits, green leafy vegetables, and fish in their meals.

Other general guidelines that will help you to have a good meal with less inflammation are:

A mix of diets: The person should always remember that there is no one food item or method to maintain good health. The body needs a variety of healthy ingredients that are practical. For an anti-inflammatory diet, the body should not be deprived of other necessary nutrients for proper functioning.

Fresh is the key: Try to buy fresh food. It does not have as much nutrition as it should if you do not eat it when it is fresh. Even if you are making your food for tomorrow, buy the foods that will stay fresh until they are eaten. There is no big difference between eating processed foods and food that has gone bad but tastes good because of what they put in it.

Check the information on labels: Before you buy food, check the label. Food can be made with sugar and fat and that is not good for your body. Some foods are already made when you buy them like cocoa which has sugar and fat in it.

Consume good-looking food: You can enjoy food even if you are curing inflammation. You can feel happy and satisfied by choosing foods you like, that will appeal to you.

Changes can be hard. When you start an anti-inflammatory diet, it might be difficult to get used to. But this change is not a big change from what you eat already. What is usually hard about this process is discipline.

Some tips that will help you to be happy when you make this process are:

Change is a slow process: When you start a new diet, do not change everything at once. Your body needs time to get used to the changes. Start slowly and then increase gradually until you are eating what you want. The same is true of snacks. We all eat too many unhealthy snacks and should replace them with healthy ones like salads with crunchy vegetables in them instead.

Choose what you love: An anti-inflammatory diet means you don't eat spicy or fried food. You should only start adding other foods to the menu if you like them too. If not, then just eat what you like. In the end, everyone is different and it's ok if they want to have rules for themselves.

Pick a variety of foods: It can be hard to eat food that doesn't taste good. If the food is ugly and doesn't look good, it can be difficult. It is better if the food looks good and you can see how fresh it is. So when you buy fruit and vegetables for your grocery cart, make sure they are colorful and look fresh too.

It is good to replace processed fast-food meals. Doing this will help you to become healthier! It's also a good idea to drink water instead of soda.

It is important to visit your doctor often. If you are suffering from chronic inflammation, you need to ask the doctor what kind of anti-inflammatory meal to have. You should also take medications and supplements if advised by the doctor.

A healthy lifestyle is important. Exercise every day and get enough sleep and you will feel better.

If you eat all natural food like fruits, vegetables, whole grains, and plant proteins, you can help avoid inflammation in your body.

Some food and drinks are bad for you. They cause inflammation. Some of those foods are processed, carbonated sugar drinks, oily food, or fried food items. Alcohol is also bad for you because it causes inflammation too.

Foods to Eat on the Anti-Inflammatory Diet

If you already eat healthy food, it should be easy to add these foods to your diet. You might already be eating them and just need to increase how much you are eating.

Some good foods that help with chronic inflammation are:

Omega 3 Fatty Acids

Omega 3 fatty acids can be found in fish and fish oil. They help calm the white blood cells, and they know there is no danger of going to sleep when they are awake. Wild salmon and other fish have these acids in them. You should try to eat three servings a week. Foods that also have Omega 3s are flax meal or dry beans such as navy beans, kidney beans, or soybeans. You can also take an Omega3 supplement if you cannot eat enough food with Omega 3s.

Fruits and Vegetables

Most fruits and vegetables are good for your body. They have lots of good things like anti-inflammatory, antioxidants, lycopene, and magnesium. These foods help make your blood cells work well.

Protective Oils and Fats

There are a few oils that you can eat if you have chronic inflammation. They are coconut oil and extra virgin olive oil. Butter or cream is also good to eat. Ghee, which is butter without the lactose and casein, is even better because it does not have these substances in them that cause trouble for people who cannot drink milk or wheat products.

Fiber

Fiber keeps waste moving through the body. There are a lot of immune cells in your intestines, so it is important to keep your gut happy. If that doesn't work, you can take a fiber supplement.

Miscellaneous

Eat foods that have healthy spices and herbs. These help your white blood cells to calm down. Spices like turmeric, cumin, cloves, ginger, and cinnamon can help. Herbs like fennel, rosemary, sage, and thyme can also reduce inflammation in your body while adding new flavors to the foods you eat.

Fermented foods like sauerkraut, buttermilk, yogurt, and kimchi have good bacteria in them that can help prevent inflammation.

Healthy snacks include yogurt with fruit, celery, carrots, pistachios, almonds and walnuts.

An example of a **GOOD** grocery list is the following :

Beans
Broccoli
Brown rice
Cabbage
Colorful and seasonal fruits
Curcumin
Fish
Green leafy vegetables
Herbs
Kale
Nuts
Oatmeal
Spices
Spinach
Turmeric
Unrefined grains with fiber
Whole-wheat bread

There are some foods that cause inflammation and you should avoid them. Foods will cause this if they are not healthy.

Processed food and sugar are two of the biggest causes of inflammation in the western diet. Processed foods are made from refined flour, so they don't have any fiber or nutrients. They contain omega 6, trans fats, and saturated fats that make inflammation worse.

Sugar is one of the worst things to eat. It hides in many foods and studies show that it can cause addictive behaviors. If you stop eating sugar, you might have a headache, cravings, and feel sluggish for a while.

Give yourself time to get better. You can still eat natural sugars a few times a week, but not too much. Eat them only at one meal per day.

Fried foods should most of the time be avoided. They are cooked in processed oils and lard, and then they are coated in flour. These things cause inflammation.

You will want to pay attention to foods that are called nightshades. Some people react negatively to these foods; if you find that you seem to have more inflammation after eating at nightshade, then it is best for you if you start changing that food in your recipes.

Instead, an example of a **BAD** grocery list (so avoid it) is the following :

Alcohol including wine
Baked goods, cookies
Eggs
Foods with added sugar or salt
Fried foods
Legumes
Margarine
Premade desserts, ice cream
Processed carbs
Processed foods
Processed meat
Processed snack foods, such as chips, crackers, and fries
Red meat
Refined carbohydrates
Soda
Sugar-sweetened beverages
Unhealthy oils
White bread, white pasta

Recipes

Breakfast

1.1 - Apple, Rhubarb and Cherries Mix

Preparation time: 10 minutes
Cooking time: 10 minutes
Servings: **4**

Ingredients:

- ½ teaspoon ginger, grated
- ½ teaspoon cinnamon powder
- 1 cup rhubarb, sliced
- 1 cup cherries, pitted and halved
- 1 apple, cored, peeled and chopped
- 2 cups almond milk
- 1 teaspoon vanilla extract

Directions:

1. Heat up a pot with the milk over medium heat, add the rhubarb, the cherries and the other ingredients, toss, cook for 10 minutes, divide into bowls and serve cold for breakfast.

Nutritional Values (Per Serving):

Calories: 200

Carbs: 13 g
Fat: 6.5 g
Fiber: 6 g
Protein: 2.3 g

Preparation time: 10 minutes
Cooking time: 20 minutes
Servings: **8**

Ingredients:

- ¼ cup coconut oil, melted
- 3 eggs, whisked
- ½ teaspoon vanilla extract
- 1 teaspoon baking powder
- 1 cup mushrooms, sliced
- ½ cup almond flour
- Cooking spray

Directions:

1. In a bowl, combine the eggs with the oil and the other ingredients, and stir well.
2. Grease a muffin tray with cooking spray, divide the mushroom mix, introduce in the oven and bake at 350 degrees F for 20 minutes.
3. Divide the muffins between plates and serve for breakfast.

Nutritional Values (Per Serving):

Calories: 167

Carbs: 15 g
Fat: 4 g
Fiber: 7 g
Protein: 6 g

1.3 - Spinach Peppers Frittata

Preparation time: 5 minutes
Cooking time: 25 minutes
Servings: **4**

Ingredients:

- 8 eggs, whisked
- ½ cup almond milk
- 1 yellow onion, chopped
- 1 tablespoon olive oil
- 1 red bell pepper, chopped
- 1 yellow bell pepper, chopped
- 1 green bell pepper, chopped
- 2 cups baby spinach
- 1 tablespoon chives, chopped
- A pinch of salt and black pepper

Directions:

1. Heat up a pan with the oil over medium-high heat, add the onion, stir and sauté for 2 minutes.
2. Add the bell peppers, stir and cook for 3 minutes more.
3. Add the eggs whisked with the milk and the other ingredients, toss, spread into the pan, introduce it in the oven and cook at 360 degrees F for 20 minutes.
4. Slice the frittata, divide it between plates and serve for breakfast.

Nutritional Values (Per Serving):

Calories: 200

Carbs: 14 g
Fat: 3 g
Fiber: 6 g
Protein: 6 g

1.4 - Almond Pancakes

Preparation time: 10 minutes
Cooking time: 10 minutes
Servings: **4**

Ingredients:

- 2 eggs, whisked
- 1 teaspoon almond extract
- 1 cup almond milk
- 2 tablespoons almonds, chopped
- 1 cup almond flour
- 2 tablespoons coconut oil, melted

Directions:

1. In a bowl, combine the eggs with the almond extract, the milk, almonds, flour and 1 tablespoon oil, and stir really well.
2. Heat up a pan with the rest of the oil over medium heat, ¼ of the batter, spread into the pan, cook for 3 minutes on each side and transfer to a plate.
3. Repeat with the rest of the batter and serve the pancakes for breakfast.

Nutritional Values (Per Serving):

Calories: 121

Carbs: 14 g
Fat: 3 g
Fiber: 6 g
Protein: 6 g

1.5 - Watermelon, Arugula and Quinoa Salad

Preparation time: 10 minutes
Cooking time: 0 minutes
Servings: **4**

Ingredients:

- ½ teaspoon maple syrup
- 2 tablespoons lemon juice
- 1 tablespoon avocado oil
- 1 cup watermelon, peeled and cubed
- 1 cup baby arugula
- 1 cup quinoa, cooked
- ½ cup basil leaves, chopped

Directions:

1. In a bowl, mix the watermelon with the arugula and the other ingredients, toss and serve for breakfast.

Nutritional Values (Per Serving):

Calories: 179

Carbs: 31.3 g
Fat: 3.2 g
Fiber: 3.4 g
Protein: 6.5 g

1.6 - Eggs with Herbs

Preparation time: 5 minutes
Cooking time: 15 minutes
Servings: **4**

Ingredients:

- 2 tablespoons olive oil
- 1 yellow onion, chopped
- 8 eggs, whisked
- A pinch of salt and black pepper
- 1 teaspoon coriander, ground
- 1 tablespoon chives, chopped
- 1 tablespoon rosemary, chopped
- 1 tablespoon cilantro, chopped
- 1 tablespoon parsley, chopped

Directions:

1. Heat up a pan with the oil over medium heat, add the onion, stir and sauté for 3 minutes.
2. Add the eggs and the other ingredients, toss, cook for 12 minutes more, divide into bowls and serve for breakfast.

Nutritional Values (Per Serving):

Calories: 200

Carbs: 3.9 g
Fat: 15.9 g
Fiber: 1 g
Protein: 11.5 g

Preparation time: 5 minutes
Cooking time: 0 minutes
Servings: **4**

Ingredients:

- 2 cups baby spinach, torn
- 2 shallots, chopped
- 1 cup cucumber, cubed
- 1 cup kalamata olives, pitted and sliced
- 1 tablespoon chives, chopped
- 1 tablespoon balsamic vinegar
- A pinch of salt and black pepper
- 2 tablespoons olive oil

Directions:

1. In a salad bowl, mix the spinach with the shallots, the cucumber and the other ingredients, toss, divide between plates and serve for breakfast.

Nutritional Values (Per Serving):

Calories: 171

Carbs: 11 g
Fat: 2 g
Fiber: 5 g
Protein: 5 g

Preparation time: 5 minutes
Cooking time: 0 minutes
Servings: **2**

Ingredients:

- 1 avocado, pitted and peeled
- 1 cup coconut milk
- 1 cup water
- 1 banana, peeled and mashed
- 1 tablespoon lime juice
- 1 cup baby spinach

Directions:

1. In your blender, combine the avocados with the milk, the water and the remaining ingredients, pulse well, divide into bowls and serve.

Nutritional Values (Per Serving):

Calories: 125

Carbs: 9 g
Fat: 6 g
Fiber: 7 g
Protein: 4 g

Preparation time: 5 minutes
Cooking time: 0 minutes
Servings: **4**

Ingredients:

- 1 cup almond milk
- 1 cup pears, cored and cubed
- 1 cup cherries, pitted and halved
- ½ teaspoon vanilla extract
- 1 tablespoon cocoa powder
- 2 tablespoons walnuts, chopped

Directions:

1. In a bowl, mix the pears with the cherries and the other ingredients, toss, divide into smaller bowls and serve for breakfast.

Nutritional Values (Per Serving):

Calories: 211

Carbs: 15.8 g
Fat: 16.9 g
Fiber: 3.4 g
Protein: 2.8 g

1.10 - Black Beans, Scallions and Eggs Mix

Preparation time: 5 minutes
Cooking time: 15 minutes
Servings: **4**

Ingredients:

- 1 cup canned black beans, drained and rinsed
- 2 green onions, chopped
- 6 eggs, whisked
- ½ teaspoon cumin, ground
- 1 teaspoon chili powder
- 2 scallions, chopped
- 1 tablespoon olive oil
- ½ cup cilantro, chopped
- 2 tablespoons pine nuts
- A pinch of salt and black pepper

Directions:

1. Heat up a pan with the oil over medium heat, add the scallions, green onions and pine nuts, stir and cook for 2 minutes.
2. Add the beans and cook them for 3 minutes more.
3. Add the eggs and the rest of the ingredients and cook for 10 minutes more, stirring often.
4. Divide everything between plates and serve for breakfast.

Nutritional Values (Per Serving):

Calories: 140

Carbs: 7 g
Fat: 4 g
Fiber: 2 g
Protein: 8 g

Lunch

Preparation time: 10 minutes
Cooking time: 12 minutes
Servings: **4**

Ingredients:

- 3 big tomatoes, cubed
- 1 pound shrimp, peeled and deveined
- 2 scallions, chopped
- 2 spring onions, chopped
- 2 tablespoons olive oil
- 1 tablespoon basil, chopped
- ½ teaspoon garlic powder
- A pinch of sea salt and white pepper
- 1 tablespoon chives, chopped

Directions:

1. Heat up a pan with the oil over medium heat, add the scallions and the spring onions, stir and sauté for 2 minutes.
2. Add the shrimp and the rest of the ingredients, toss, cook over medium heat for 10 minutes, divide into bowls and serve for lunch.

Nutritional Values (Per Serving):

Calories: 200

Carbs: 14 g
Fat: 4 g
Fiber: 6 g
Protein: 9 g

Preparation time: 10 minutes
Cooking time: 30 minutes
Servings: **4**

Ingredients:

- 1 yellow onion, chopped
- 2 tablespoons olive oil
- 2 garlic cloves, minced
- 1 pound chicken thighs, skinless, boneless and cubed ½ teaspoon turmeric powder ½ teaspoon red chili flakes
- A pinch of salt and black pepper
- 6 cups veggie stock
- 1 bunch chard, roughly chopped
- 1 tablespoon cilantro, chopped

Directions:

1. Heat up a pot with the oil over medium heat, add the onion and the garlic and sauté for 5 minutes.
2. Add the meat and brown for 5 minutes more.
3. Add the stock and the other ingredients, toss, bring to a simmer and cook over medium heat for 20 minutes more.
4. Divide the soup into bowls and serve.

Nutritional Values (Per Serving):

Calories: 181

Carbs: 9 g
Fat: 4 g
Fiber: 4 g
Protein: 11 g

Preparation time: 10 minutes
Cooking time: 0 minutes
Servings: **4**

Ingredients:

- 1 pound smoked salmon, skinless, boneless and cut into strips
- 2 cucumbers, peeled and cubed
- 1 pineapple, peeled and cubed
- 1 tablespoon balsamic vinegar
- 2 tablespoons olive oil
- 1 tablespoon cilantro, chopped
- A pinch of salt and black pepper

Directions:

1. In a salad bowl, mix the salmon with the cucumbers, the pineapple and the other ingredients, toss and serve for lunch.

Nutritional Values (Per Serving):

Calories: 327

Carbs: 10. 9 g
Fat: 12.2 g
Fiber: 1.4 g
Protein: 21.9 g

2.4 - Lemon Shrimp with Zucchini

Preparation time: 10 minutes
Cooking time: 17 minutes
Servings: **4**

Ingredients:

- 1 pound shrimp, peeled and deveined
- 1 tablespoon lemon juice
- 2 zucchinis, sliced
- 1 yellow onion, roughly chopped
- 1 tablespoon olive oil
- 1 teaspoon turmeric powder
- A pinch of salt and black pepper
- 1 tablespoons capers, drained
- 2 tablespoons pine nuts

Directions:

1. Heat up a pan with the oil over medium-high heat, add the onion and the zucchini, stir and sauté for 5 minutes.
2. Add the shrimp and the other ingredients, toss, cook everything for 12 minutes more, divide into bowls and serve for lunch.

Nutritional Values (Per Serving):

Calories: 162

Carbs: 12 g
Fat: 3 g
Fiber: 4 g
Protein: 7 g

Preparation time: 5 minutes
Cooking time: 30 minutes
Servings: **4**

Ingredients:

- ½ pound cauliflower florets
- 1 pound cod fillets, boneless, skinless and cubed
- 1 tablespoon olive oil
- 1 yellow onion, chopped
- ½ teaspoon cumin seeds
- 1 green chili, chopped
- ¼ teaspoon turmeric powder
- 2 tomatoes chopped
- A pinch of salt and black pepper
- ½ cup chicken stock
- 1 tablespoon cilantro, chopped

Directions:

1. Heat up a pot with the oil over medium heat, add the onion, chili, cumin and turmeric, stir and cook for 5 minutes.
2. Add the cauliflower, the fish and the other ingredients, toss, bring to a simmer and cook over medium heat for 25 minutes more.
3. Divide the stew into bowls and serve.

Nutritional Values (Per Serving):

Calories: 281

Carbs: 8 g
Fat: 6 g
Fiber: 4 g
Protein: 12 g

Preparation time: 10 minutes
Cooking time: 45 minutes
Servings: **4**

Ingredients:

- 1 tablespoon olive oil
- 1 pound chicken thighs, skinless, boneless and cubed
- 2 garlic cloves, minced
- 1 small yellow onion, chopped
- 1 green bell pepper, chopped
- 1 red bell pepper, chopped
- ½ teaspoon cumin, ground
- ½ teaspoon sweet paprika
- 2 cups chicken stock
- A pinch of salt and black pepper
- 1 tablespoon lemon juice
- 1 cup coconut milk
- 1 tablespoon cilantro, chopped

Directions:

1. Heat up a pot with the oil over medium heat, add the onion, garlic and the meat and brown for 10 minutes stirring often.
2. Add the rest of the ingredients except the coconut milk and the cilantro, stir, bring to a simmer and cook over medium for 30 minutes more.
3. Add the coconut milk and the cilantro, stir, simmer the stew for 5 minutes more, divide into bowls and serve for lunch.

Calories: 419

Carbs: 10.7 g
Fat: 26.8 g
Fiber: 2.7 g
Protein: 35.5 g

2.7 - Chili Turkey Meatballs

Preparation time: 10 minutes
Cooking time: 10 minutes
Servings: **4**

Ingredients:

- 1 pound turkey meat, ground
- 1 yellow onion, chopped
- 1 egg, whisked
- 1 tablespoon cilantro, chopped
- 2 tablespoons olive oil
- 1 red chili pepper, minced
- 2 teaspoons lime juice
- Zest of 1 lime, grated
- A pinch of salt and black pepper
- 1 teaspoon turmeric powder

Directions:

1. In a bowl, combine the turkey meat with the onion and the other ingredients except the oil, stir and shape medium meatballs out of this mix.
2. Heat up a pan with the oil over medium-high heat, add the meatballs, cook them for 5 minutes on each side, divide between plates and serve for lunch.

Nutritional Values (Per Serving):

Calories: 200

Carbs: 12 g
Fat: 12 g
Fiber: 5 g
Protein: 7 g

Preparation time: 10 minutes
Cooking time: 15 minutes
Servings: **4**

Ingredients:

- 1 yellow onion, chopped
- 1 tablespoon olive oil
- 1 pound salmon fillets, boneless and cubed
- 2 teaspoons horseradish
- ¼ cup coconut cream
- A pinch of salt and black pepper
- ½ teaspoon sweet paprika
- 1 teaspoon cumin, ground
- 1 tablespoon chives, chopped

Directions:

1. Heat up a pan with the oil over medium heat, add the onion and the fish and cook for 5 minutes.
2. Add the rest of the ingredients, toss, cook everything for 10 minutes more, divide into bowls and serve for lunch.

Nutritional Values (Per Serving):

Calories: 233

Carbs: 9 g
Fat: 6 g
Fiber: 5 g
Protein: 9 g

2.9 - Chili Mushroom Stew

Preparation time: 5 minutes
Cooking time: 30 minutes
Servings: **4**

Ingredients:

- 1 yellow onion, chopped
- 1 tablespoon olive oil
- 1 pound white mushrooms, sliced
- 1 cup chicken stock
- 1 cup tomato puree
- 1 carrot, sliced
- 1 teaspoon turmeric powder
- 1 teaspoon chili powder
- ½ teaspoon cumin, ground
- 1 teaspoon coriander, ground
- 2 garlic cloves, minced
- A pinch of salt and black pepper
- 1 tablespoon cilantro, chopped

Directions:

1. Heat up a pot with the oil over medium heat, add the onion and the mushrooms, stir and sauté for 5 minutes.
2. Add the carrot and the garlic and cook for 5 minutes more.
3. Add the stock and the other ingredients except the cilantro, stir, bring to a simmer and cook over medium heat for 20 minutes.
4. Divide the stew into bowls, sprinkle the cilantro on top and serve.

Nutritional Values (Per Serving):

Calories: 199

Carbs: 14 g
Fat: 4 g
Fiber: 6 g
Protein: 7 g

Preparation time: 5 minutes
Cooking time: 20 minutes
Servings: **4**

Ingredients:

- 4 sea bass fillets, boneless
- 1 yellow onion, chopped
- 2 tablespoons olive oil
- 1 tablespoon lemon juice
- 1 tablespoon oregano, chopped
- 2 garlic cloves, chopped
- Salt and black pepper to the taste
- 1 cup cherry tomatoes, halved
- 1 tablespoon chives, chopped

Directions:

1. Heat up a pan with the oil over medium heat, add the onion and the garlic and sauté for 2 minutes.
2. Add the fish and sear it for 2 minutes on each side.
3. Add the rest of the ingredients, cook everything for 14 minutes more, divide between plates and serve.

Nutritional Values (Per Serving):

Calories: 273

Carbs: 10 g
Fat: 6 g
Fiber: 6 g
Protein: 11 g

Preparation time: 10 minutes
Cooking time: 20 minutes
Servings: **4**

Ingredients:

- 1 pound shrimp, peeled and deveined
- 4 scallions, chopped
- 1 teaspoon sweet paprika
- 1 tablespoon olive oil
- Juice of 1 lime
- Zest of 1 lime, grated
- A pinch of salt and black pepper
- 2 tablespoons parsley, chopped

Directions:

1. Heat up a pan with the oil over medium heat, add the scallions and sauté for 5 minutes.
2. Add the shrimp and the other ingredients, toss, cook over medium heat for 15 minutes more, divide into bowls and serve.

Nutritional Values (Per Serving):

Calories: 172

Carbs: 3.3 g
Fat: 5.5 g
Fiber: 0.7 g
Protein: 26.2 g

Side Dishes

Preparation time: 10 minutes
Cooking time: 20 minutes
Servings: **4**

Ingredients:

- 1 pound mushrooms, sliced
- 1 yellow onion, chopped
- 1 tablespoon ginger, grated
- 1 tablespoon olive oil
- 2 tablespoons balsamic vinegar
- 2 garlic cloves, minced
- A pinch of salt and black pepper
- ¼ cup lime juice
- 2 tablespoons walnuts, chopped

Directions:

1. Heat up a pan with the oil over medium-high heat, add the onion and the ginger and sauté for 5 minutes.
2. Add the mushrooms and the other ingredients, toss, cook over medium heat for 15 minutes more, divide between plates and serve.

Nutritional Values (Per Serving):

Calories: 120

Carbs: 4 g
Fat: 2 g
Fiber: 2 g
Protein: 5 g

Preparation time: 5 minutes
Cooking time: 0 minutes
Servings: **4**

Ingredients:

- 2 cups barley, cooked
- 1 cup baby kale
- 2 tablespoons almonds, chopped
- 2 tablespoons balsamic vinegar
- 1 tablespoon olive oil
- 1 tablespoon cilantro, chopped

Directions:

1. In a bowl, mix the barley with the kale, the almonds and the other ingredients, toss and serve as a side dish.

Nutritional Values (Per Serving):

Calories: 175

Carbs: 5 g
Fat: 3 g
Fiber: 3 g
Protein: 6 g

Preparation time: 10 minutes
Cooking time: 0 minutes
Servings: **4**

Ingredients:

- 1 cup quinoa, cooked
- 1 cup baby spinach
- A pinch of sea salt and black pepper
- 1 cucumber, chopped
- 1 teaspoon chili powder
- 2 tablespoons balsamic vinegar
- 2 tablespoons cilantro, chopped

Directions:

1. In a bowl, mix the quinoa with the spinach and the other ingredients, toss and serve as a side dish.

Nutritional Values (Per Serving):

Calories: 100

Carbs: 6 g
Fat: 0.5 g
Fiber: 2 g
Protein: 6 g

Preparation time: 10 minutes
Cooking time: 20 minutes
Servings: **4**

Ingredients:

- 1 pound broccoli florets
- 1 cup green peas
- 1 teaspoon cumin, ground
- A pinch of salt and black pepper
- 1 tablespoon mint leaves, chopped
- 2 tablespoons olive oil
- 1 tablespoon coriander, chopped

Directions:

1. In a roasting pan, combine the broccoli with the peas, the mint and the other ingredients, toss and bake at 390 degrees F for 20 minutes.
2. Divide everything between plates and serve.

Nutritional Values (Per Serving):

Calories: 120

Carbs: 5 g
Fat: 6 g
Fiber: 1 g
Protein: 6 g

3.5 - Cabbage and Dates Salad

Preparation time: 10 minutes
Cooking time: 0 minutes
Servings: **4**

Ingredients:

- 2 cups green cabbage, shredded
- 1 carrot, grated
- 4 dates, chopped
- 2 tablespoons walnuts, chopped
- 1 tablespoon lemon juice
- 2 garlic cloves, minced
- 1 tablespoon apple cider vinegar
- 3 tablespoons olive oil
- 1 tablespoon parsley, chopped
- A pinch of salt and black pepper

Directions:

1. In a bowl, combine the cabbage with the carrots, dates and the other ingredients, toss and serve as a side salad.

Nutritional Values (Per Serving):

Calories: 140

Carbs: 5 g
Fat: 3 g
Fiber: 4 g
Protein: 14 g

3.6 - Rice and Tomato Mix

Preparation time: 10 minutes
Cooking time: 0 minutes
Servings: **4**

Ingredients:

- 2 tablespoons olive oil
- 2 cups brown rice, cooked
- ½ cup cherry tomatoes, halved
- 2 teaspoons cumin, ground
- ¼ cup cilantro, chopped
- A pinch of salt and black pepper
- 2 tablespoons olive oil

Directions:

1. In a bowl, combine the rice with the oil and the other ingredients, toss and serve.

Nutritional Values (Per Serving):

Calories: 122

Carbs: 8 g
Fat: 4 g
Fiber: 3 g
Protein: 5 g

Preparation time: 10 minutes
Cooking time: 25 minutes
Servings: **4**

Ingredients:

- 1 pound mushrooms, sliced
- 1 yellow onion, chopped
- 1 teaspoon cumin, ground
- 1 teaspoon sweet paprika
- 1 cup canned black beans, drained and rinsed
- 2 tablespoons olive oil
- ½ cup chicken stock
- A pinch of salt and black pepper
- 2 tablespoons cilantro, chopped

Directions:

1. Heat up a pan with the oil over medium heat, add the onion and sauté for 5 minutes.
2. Add the mushrooms and sauté for 5 minutes more.
3. Add the rest of the ingredients, toss, cook over medium heat for 15 minutes more.
4. Divide everything between plates and serve as a side dish.

Calories: 189

Carbs: 9 g
Fat: 3 g
Fiber: 4 g
Protein: 8 g

Preparation time: 5 minutes
Cooking time: 0 minutes
Servings: **4**

Ingredients:

- 2 cucumbers, sliced
- 1 green apple, cored and cubed
- 3 spring onions, chopped
- 3 tablespoons olive oil
- 4 teaspoons orange juice
- A pinch of salt and black pepper
- 1 tablespoon mint, chopped
- 1 tablespoon lemon juice

Directions:

1. In a bowl, mix the cucumbers with the apple, spring onions and the other ingredients, toss and serve as a side salad.

Nutritional Values (Per Serving):

Calories: 110

Carbs: 6 g
Fat: 0 g
Fiber: 3 g
Protein: 8 g

Preparation time: 5 minutes
Cooking time: 15 minutes
Servings: **4**

Ingredients:

- 3 endives, shredded
- 1 tablespoon olive oil
- 4 scallions, chopped
- ½ cup tomato sauce
- 2 garlic cloves, minced
- A pinch of sea salt and black pepper
- 1/8 teaspoon turmeric powder
- 1 tablespoon chives, chopped

Directions:

1. Heat up a pan with the oil over medium heat, add the scallions and the garlic and sauté for 5 minutes.
2. Add the endives and the other ingredients, toss, cook everything for 10 minutes more, divide between plates and serve as a side dish.

Nutritional Values (Per Serving):

Calories: 110

Carbs: 16.2 g
Fat: 4.4 g
Fiber: 12.8 g
Protein: 5.6 g

Preparation time: 10 minutes
Cooking time: 25 minutes
Servings: **4**

Ingredients:

- 1 pound cauliflower florets
- 2 tablespoons avocado oil
- 1 teaspoon nutmeg, ground
- 1 teaspoon hot paprika
- 1 tablespoon pumpkin seeds
- 1 tablespoon chives, chopped
- A pinch of sea salt and black pepper

Directions:

1. Spread the cauliflower florets on a baking sheet lined with parchment paper, add the oil, the nutmeg and the other ingredients, toss and bake at 380 degrees F for 25 minutes.
2. Divide the cauliflower mix between plates and serve as a side dish.

Nutritional Values (Per Serving):

Calories: 160

Carbs: 9 g
Fat: 3 g
Fiber: 2 g
Protein: 4 g

3.11 - Walnut Sprouts Mix

Preparation time: 5 minutes
Cooking time: 30 minutes
Servings: **4**

Ingredients:

- 1 pound Brussels sprouts, trimmed and halved
- 2 carrots, grated
- 2 tablespoons avocado oil
- 1 tablespoon rosemary, chopped
- 2 tablespoons walnuts, chopped
- A pinch of salt and black pepper

Directions:

1. In a baking dish, mix the sprouts with the carrots, the oil and the other ingredients, toss and bake at 380 degrees F for 30 minutes.
2. Divide everything between plates and serve as a side dish.

Nutritional Values (Per Serving):

Calories: 191

Carbs: 13 g
Fat: 2 g
Fiber: 4 g
Protein: 7 g

Snacks

Preparation time: 10 minutes
Cooking time: 15 minutes
Servings: **4**

Ingredients:

- ½ cup sunflower seeds
- ½ cup chia seeds
- ½ cup pine nuts
- ½ cup pumpkin seeds
- 1 tablespoon coconut oil, melted
- 1 teaspoon sweet paprika

Directions:

1. Spread the seeds on a baking sheet lined with parchment paper, add the oil and the paprika, toss and cook for 15 minutes at 400 degrees F.
2. Divide into bowls and serve.

Nutritional Values (Per Serving):

Calories: 110

Carbs: 7 g
Fat: 1 g
Fiber: 5 g
Protein: 5 g

Preparation time: 10 minutes
Cooking time: 20 minutes
Servings: **8**

Ingredients:

- 1 garlic head, peeled and cloves separated
- 1 cup coconut cream
- 1 cup spinach, torn
- 1 tablespoon olive oil
- 1 teaspoon rosemary, dried
- 1 tablespoon chives, chopped
- A pinch of salt and black pepper

Directions:

1. Heat up a pan with the oil over medium heat, add the garlic and sauté for 10 minutes.
2. Add the spinach, cream and the other ingredients, whisk, cook over medium heat for 10 minutes more, blend using an immersion blender, divide into bowls and serve.

Nutritional Values (Per Serving):

Calories: 100

Carbs: 8 g
Fat: 3 g
Fiber: 4 g
Protein: 5 g

Preparation time: 10 minutes
Cooking time: 15 minutes
Servings: **4**

Ingredients:

- 2 tablespoons olive oil
- 1 pound kale leaves, pat dried
- 2 tablespoons garlic, minced
- 1 tablespoon lemon zest, grated
- Salt and black pepper to the taste

Directions:

1. Spread the kale leaves on a baking sheet lined with parchment paper, add the oil and the other ingredients, toss a bit and cook in the oven at 400 degrees F for 15 minutes.
2. Cool the kale chips down, divide into bowls and serve as a snack.

Nutritional Values (Per Serving):

Calories: 149

Carbs: 9 g
Fat: 4 g
Fiber: 3 g
Protein: 6 g

Preparation time: 10 minutes
Cooking time: 0 minutes
Servings: **4**

Ingredients:

- 2 cups pineapple, peeled and cubed
- 4 scallions, chopped
- ¼ cup cilantro, chopped
- 1 green chili pepper, chopped
- 2 tomatoes, cubed
- 2 tablespoons olive oil
- Salt and black pepper to the taste
- 1 tablespoon lemon juice
- A pinch cayenne pepper

Directions:

1. In a bowl, combine the pineapple with the scallions and the other ingredients, toss well and serve as a party salsa.

Nutritional Values (Per Serving):

Calories: 100

Carbs: 8 g
Fat: 3.8 g
Fiber: 4 g
Protein: 9 g

4.5 - Baked Walnut Snack

Preparation time: 10 minutes
Cooking time: 14 minutes
Servings: **4**

Ingredients:

- 1 cup walnuts
- 1 tablespoon olive oil
- 1 teaspoon garlic powder
- 1 teaspoon smoked paprika
- A pinch of salt and black pepper

Directions:

1. Spread the walnuts on a baking sheet lined with parchment paper, add the oil and the other ingredients, toss and bake at 400 degrees F for 14 minutes.
2. Divide the mix into bowls and serve.

Nutritional Values (Per Serving):

Calories: 100

Carbs: 11 g
Fat: 2 g
Fiber: 4 g
Protein: 6 g

Preparation time: 10 minutes
Cooking time: 25 minutes
Servings: **4**

Ingredients:

- 1 pound broccoli florets
- Cooking spray
- 2 eggs, whisked
- 1 teaspoon Italian seasoning
- A pinch of sea salt and black pepper
- 1 teaspoon smoked paprika
- 1 teaspoon cumin, ground

Directions:

1. In a bowl, mix the eggs with the Italian seasoning and the other ingredients except the broccoli and the cooking spray and whisk well.
2. Dip the broccoli florets in the eggs mix, arrange them on a baking sheet lined with parchment paper, grease them with cooking spray and bake at 380 degrees F for 25 minutes.
3. Divide the broccoli bites into bowls and serve.

Nutritional Values (Per Serving):

Calories: 120

Carbs: 6 g
Fat: 6 g
Fiber: 2 g
Protein: 7 g

Preparation time: 10 minutes
Cooking time: 20 minutes
Servings: **6**

Ingredients:

- 2 cups canned red kidney beans, drained
- 2 tablespoons olive oil
- 1 yellow onion, chopped
- ½ cup chicken stock
- ½ cup coconut cream
- ¼ teaspoon oregano, dried
- ¼ teaspoon garlic powder
- ¼ teaspoon onion powder
- Salt and black pepper to the taste
- 1 tablespoon chives, chopped

Directions:

---

1. Heat up a pan with the oil over medium heat, add the onion and sauté for 5 minutes.
2. Add the stock, oregano and the other ingredients except the cream and the chives, stir, and cook over medium heat for 15 minutes more.
3. Add the cream, blend the mix using an immersion blender, divide into bowls and serve with the chives sprinkled on top.

Nutritional Values (Per Serving):

Calories: 302

Carbs: 40.7 g
Fat: 10.2 g
Fiber: 10.2 g
Protein: 14.6 g

Preparation time: 10 minutes
Cooking time: 12 minutes
Servings: **6**

Ingredients:

- 1 pound tomatoes, chopped
- 2 carrots, grated
- 4 ounces coconut cream
- A pinch of salt and black pepper
- 1 teaspoon chili powder
- Cooking spray

Directions:

1. In a pan, combine the tomatoes with the carrots and the other ingredients, toss and cook over medium heat for 12 minutes.
2. Blend using an immersion blender, divide into small bowls and serve as a party dip.

Nutritional Values (Per Serving):

Calories: 150

Carbs: 14 g
Fat: 4 g
Fiber: 6 g
Protein: 6 g

Preparation time: 10 minutes
Cooking time: 15 minutes
Servings: **4**

Ingredients:

- 4 celery stalks
- 3 scallions, chopped
- 1 tablespoon olive oil
- 1 tablespoon lime juice
- ½ teaspoon chili powder
- 1 cup coconut cream
- Salt and black pepper to the taste
- 2 tablespoons parsley, chopped

Directions:

1. Heat up a pan with the oil over medium heat, add the scallions and sauté for 2 minutes.
2. Add the celery and the other ingredients, toss, cook over medium heat for 13 minutes more, blend using an immersion blender, divide into bowls and serve s a snack.

Nutritional Values (Per Serving):

Calories: 140

Carbs: 6 g
Fat: 10 g
Fiber: 3 g
Protein: 13 g

Preparation time: 10 minutes
Cooking time: 25 minutes
Servings: **8**

Ingredients:

- 1 tablespoon olive oil
- 1 yellow onion, chopped
- 1 pound white mushrooms, sliced
- 1 teaspoon turmeric powder
- 1 teaspoon coriander, ground
- 3 garlic cloves, minced
- 2 cups coconut cream
- A pinch of salt and black pepper
- 1 tablespoon dill, chopped

Directions:

1. Heat up a pan with the oil over medium heat, add the onion and the garlic and sauté for 5 minutes.
2. Add the mushrooms and sauté for 5 minutes more.
3. Add the rest of the ingredients, stir, cook over medium heat for 15 minutes, blend using an immersion blender, divide into bowls and serve.

Nutritional Values (Per Serving):

Calories: 120

Carbs: 10 g
Fat: 8 g
Fiber: 5 g
Protein: 9 g

Poultry

Preparation time: 5 minutes
Cooking time: 35 minutes
Servings: **4**

Ingredients:

- 2 pounds chicken thighs, skinless, boneless and cubed
- 1 yellow onion, chopped
- 2 tablespoons olive oil
- A pinch of salt and black pepper
- 1 cup baby spinach
- 1 fennel bulb, sliced
- ½ teaspoon fennel seeds, crushed
- ½ teaspoon coriander, ground
- ½ cup chicken stock
- 1 tablespoon cilantro, chopped
- 1 tablespoon chives, chopped

Directions:

1. Heat up a pan with the oil over medium-high heat, add the onion and the fennel and sauté for 5 minutes.
2. Add the chicken and brown for 5 minutes more.
3. Add the fennel seeds and the other ingredients, toss, bring to a simmer and cook over medium heat for 25 minutes more.
4. Divide the mix between plates and serve.

Nutritional Values (Per Serving):

Calories: 288

Carbs: 12 g
Fat: 4 g
Fiber: 6 g
Protein: 7 g

Preparation time: 10 minutes
Cooking time: 40 minutes
Servings: **4**

Ingredients:

- 1 pound turkey breast, skinless, boneless and sliced
- 1 cup quinoa
- 3 cups chicken stock
- ½ cup radish, sliced
- 2 tablespoons olive oil
- A pinch of salt and black pepper
- 4 scallions, chopped
- ¼ cup basil, torn

Directions:

1. Heat up a pan with the oil over medium-high heat, add the scallions and the meat and brown for 5 minutes.
2. Add the quinoa and the other ingredients, toss, bring to a simmer and cook over medium heat for 35 minutes.
3. Divide everything between plates and serve.

Nutritional Values (Per Serving):

Calories: 213

Carbs: 9 g
Fat: 3 g
Fiber: 5 g
Protein: 6 g

Preparation time: 10 minutes
Cooking time: 30 minutes
Servings: **4**

Ingredients:

- 1 yellow onion, chopped
- 2 tablespoons olive oil
- 1 pound chicken breast, skinless, boneless and sliced
- 1 cup peaches, peeled and cubed
- 3 tablespoons lime juice
- A pinch of salt and black pepper
- 1 tablespoon lime zest, grated
- 1 tablespoon cilantro, chopped

Directions:

1. Heat up a pan with the oil over medium-high heat, add the onion and sauté for 5 minutes.
2. Add the meat and brown for 5 minutes more.
3. Add the rest of the ingredients, toss, cook over medium heat for 20 minutes, divide between plates and serve.

Nutritional Values (Per Serving):

Calories: 271

Carbs: 16 g
Fat: 4 g
Fiber: 8 g
Protein: 8 g

Preparation time: 10 minutes
Cooking time: 1 hour
Servings: **4**

Ingredients:

- 2 cups canned chickpeas, drained and rinsed
- 2 pounds chicken breast, skinless, boneless and sliced
- 1 cup chicken stock
- A pinch of salt and black pepper
- 1 teaspoon cumin, ground
- 1 teaspoon sweet paprika
- 1 teaspoon coriander, ground
- 2 tablespoons avocado oil
- 1 yellow onion, chopped
- 2 red bell peppers, chopped
- 1 tablespoon garlic powder
- 1 tablespoon chives, chopped

Directions:

1. Heat up a pan with the oil over medium heat, add the onion and the meat and brown for 5 minutes.
2. Add the chickpeas and the other ingredients, toss, introduce in the oven at 350 degrees F, bake for 55 minutes, divide between plates and serve.

Nutritional Values (Per Serving):

Calories: 244

Carbs: 10 g
Fat: 11 g
Fiber: 4 g
Protein: 13 g

Preparation time: 10 minutes
Cooking time: 40 minutes
Servings: **4**

Ingredients:

- 2 pounds chicken breasts, skinless, boneless and cubed
- 1 cup canned black beans, drained and rinsed
- 1 cup canned red kidney beans, drained and rinsed
- 1 yellow onion, chopped
- 2 tablespoons avocado oil
- A pinch of salt and black pepper
- 1 teaspoon smoked paprika
- 1 teaspoon basil, dried
- 1 cup chicken stock
- 1 cup canned tomatoes, crushed
- 1 tablespoon parsley, chopped

Directions:

1. Heat up a pan with the oil over medium-high heat, add the onion and sauté for 5 minutes.
2. Add the meat and brown it for 5 minutes more.
3. Add the beans and the other ingredients, toss, reduce heat to medium and cook everything for 30 minutes more.
4. Divide the mix between plates and serve.

Nutritional Values (Per Serving):

Calories: 312

Carbs: 15 g
Fat: 7 g
Fiber: 7 g
Protein: 15 g

Preparation time: 10 minutes
Cooking time: 8 hours
Servings: **6**

Ingredients:

- 2 pounds chicken breast, skinless, boneless and sliced
- 2 tablespoons olive oil
- 2 cups corn
- 2 teaspoons garlic powder
- A pinch of salt and black pepper
- 2 cups coconut milk
- 2 tablespoons parsley, chopped
- 3 green onions, chopped

Directions:

1. In your slow cooker, combine the chicken with the oil, the corn and the other ingredients, toss, put the lid on and cook on Low for 8 hours.
2. Divide everything between plates and serve.

Nutritional Values (Per Serving):

Calories: 265

Carbs: 10 g
Fat: 8 g
Fiber: 10 g
Protein: 24 g

Preparation time: 10 minutes
Cooking time: 40 minutes
Servings: **4**

Ingredients:

- 1 yellow onion, chopped
- 5 garlic cloves, minced
- 1 tablespoon orange juice
- 2 tablespoons olive oil
- 1 tablespoon orange zest, grated
- 1 cup chicken stock
- 1 pound chicken breast, skinless, boneless and cubed A pinch of salt and black pepper
- 1 cup baby spinach
- 1 teaspoon cumin, ground
- 1 tablespoon cilantro, chopped

Directions:

1. Heat up a pan with the oil over medium heat, add the onion and the garlic and sauté for 5 minutes.
2. Add the meat, orange juice and zest and brown for 5 minutes more.
3. Add the rest of the ingredients, toss, cook over medium heat for 30 minutes, divide between plates and serve.

Nutritional Values (Per Serving):

Calories: 250

Carbs: 14 g
Fat: 3 g
Fiber: 3 g
Protein: 7 g

Preparation time: 10 minutes
Cooking time: 1 hour
Servings: **4**

Ingredients:

- 2 pounds turkey breast, skinless, boneless and sliced
- 2 tablespoons avocado oil
- 1 yellow onion, sliced
- 2 spring onions, chopped
- A pinch of salt and black pepper
- 1 cup chicken stock
- 2 teaspoons lemon juice
- 1 teaspoon coriander, ground

Directions:

1. In a roasting pan, combine the turkey with the oil, the onion and the other ingredients, toss and bake at 390 degrees F for 1 hour.
2. Divide the mix between plates and serve.

Nutritional Values (Per Serving):

Calories: 300

Carbs: 15 g
Fat: 4 g
Fiber: 4 g
Protein: 27 g

Preparation time: 10 minutes
Cooking time: 0 minutes
Servings: **4**

Ingredients:

- 2 cups rotisserie chicken, cooked and shredded
- 1 cup tomatoes, cubed
- 1 cucumber, sliced
- 1 yellow onion, chopped
- 2 tablespoons olive oil
- 1 tablespoon lemon juice
- Salt and black pepper to the taste
- 1 tablespoon chives, chopped

Directions:

1. In a salad bowl, combine the chicken with the tomatoes, the cucumber and the other ingredients, toss and serve.

Nutritional Values (Per Serving):

Calories: 234

Carbs: 12 g
Fat: 8 g
Fiber: 4 g
Protein: 15 g

Preparation time: 5 minutes
Cooking time: 40 minutes
Servings: **4**

Ingredients:

- 2 pounds chicken thighs, boneless, skinless
- 2 tablespoons olive oil
- 4 scallions, chopped
- 2 sweet potatoes, peeled and cut into wedges
- 1 tablespoon lemon juice
- 1 teaspoon coriander, ground
- A pinch of salt and black pepper
- 1 tablespoon ginger, minced
- 1 tablespoon rosemary, chopped

Directions:

---

1. Heat up a pan with the oil over medium-high heat, add the scallions, ginger and the meat and brown for 10 minutes stirring often.
2. Add the rest of the ingredients, toss, cook over medium heat for 30 minutes more, divide between plates and serve.

Nutritional Values (Per Serving):

Calories: 210

Carbs: 12 g
Fat: 8 g
Fiber: 4 g
Protein: 17 g

Meat

6.1 - Cinnamon Pork Mix

Preparation time: 10 minutes
Cooking time: 1 hour
Servings: **4**

Ingredients:

- 2 pounds pork stew meat, cubed
- 2 tablespoons olive oil
- 1 yellow onion, chopped
- 2 avocados, peeled, pitted and sliced
- 1 tablespoon chili powder
- Salt and black pepper to the taste
- 1 teaspoon cumin, ground
- ½ teaspoon cinnamon powder
- A pinch of cayenne pepper
- ½ cup vegetable stock
- ½ cup parsley, chopped

Directions:

1. Heat up a pan with the oil over medium-high heat, add the onion and the meat and brown for 10 minutes stirring often.
2. Add the avocados and the other ingredients, toss, introduce the pan in the oven and bake at 390 degrees F for 50 minutes.
3. Divide the mix between plates and serve.

Nutritional Values (Per Serving):

Calories: 300

Carbs: 12 g
Fat: 7 g
Fiber: 6 g
Protein: 18 g

Preparation time: 10 minutes
Cooking time: 35 minutes
Servings: **4**

Ingredients:

- 2 tablespoons balsamic vinegar
- 1 cup canned artichoke hearts, drained and quartered
- 2 tablespoons olive oil
- 2 pounds pork stew meat, cubed
- 2 tablespoons parsley, chopped
- 1 teaspoon cumin, ground
- 1 teaspoon turmeric powder
- 2 garlic cloves, minced
- A pinch of sea salt and black pepper

Directions:

1. Heat up a pan with the oil over medium heat, add the meat and brown for 5 minutes.
2. Add the artichokes, the vinegar and the other ingredients, toss, cook over medium heat for 30 minutes, divide between plates and serve.

Nutritional Values (Per Serving):

Calories: 260

Carbs: 11 g
Fat: 5 g
Fiber: 4 g
Protein: 20 g

Preparation time: 10 minutes
Cooking time: 40 minutes
Servings: **4**

Ingredients:

- 2 pounds pork stew meat, cut into strips
- ½ cup corn
- ½ cup green peas
- 2 tablespoons olive oil
- ½ cup yellow onion, chopped
- 3 tablespoons coconut aminos
- ½ cup vegetable stock
- A pinch of salt and black pepper

Directions:

1. Heat up a pan with the oil over medium heat, add the meat and the onion and brown for 10 minutes.
2. Add the corn and the other ingredients, toss, cook over medium heat for 30 minutes more, divide between plates and serve.

Nutritional Values (Per Serving):

Calories: 250

Carbs: 9.7 g
Fat: 4 g
Fiber: 6 g
Protein: 12 g

Preparation time: 5 minutes
Cooking time: 1 hour
Servings: **4**

Ingredients:

- 2 tablespoons olive oil
- 2 pounds pork chops
- 4 scallions, chopped
- A pinch of salt and black pepper
- 2 garlic cloves, minced
- ¼ cup chicken stock
- 1 cup tomato sauce
- 2 tablespoons lime juice
- 1 tablespoon herbs de Provence

Directions:

1. Heat up a pan with the oil over medium heat, add the scallions and the garlic and sauté for 5 minutes.
2. Add the meat and brown for 5 minutes more.
3. Add the remaining ingredients, toss and bake everything at 380 degrees F for 50 minutes.
4. Divide the whole mix between plates and serve.

Nutritional Values (Per Serving):

Calories: 251

Carbs: 9 g
Fat: 3 g
Fiber: 6 g
Protein: 16 g

Preparation time: 10 minutes
Cooking time: 1 hour
Servings: **4**

Ingredients:

- 2 pounds pork roast, sliced
- 2 sweet potatoes, peeled and sliced
- 2 tablespoons olive oil
- 1 teaspoon rosemary, dried
- 1 teaspoon turmeric powder
- 2 yellow onions, sliced
- ½ cup veggie stock
- A pinch of salt and black pepper

Directions:

1. In a roasting pan, combine the pork slices with the sweet potatoes, the onions and the other ingredients, toss and bake at 400 degrees F for 1 hours.
2. Divide everything between plates and serve.

Nutritional Values (Per Serving):

Calories: 290

Carbs: 10 g
Fat: 4 g
Fiber: 7 g
Protein: 17 g

Preparation time: 5 minutes
Cooking time: 10 minutes
Servings: **4**

Ingredients:

- 1 pound pork stew meat, cut into strips
- 3 tablespoons olive oil
- 4 scallions, chopped
- 2 tablespoons lemon juice
- 2 tablespoons balsamic vinegar
- 2 cups mixed salad greens
- 1 avocado, peeled, pitted and roughly cubed
- 1 cucumber, sliced
- 2 tomatoes, cubed
- A pinch of salt and black pepper

Directions:

1. Heat up a pan with 2 tablespoons of oil over medium heat, add the scallions, the meat and the lemon juice, toss and cook for 10 minutes.
2. In a salad bowl, combine the salad greens with the meat and the remaining ingredients, toss and serve.

Nutritional Values (Per Serving):

Calories: 225

Carbs: 8 g
Fat: 6.4 g
Fiber: 4 g
Protein: 11 g

Preparation time: 10 minutes
Cooking time: 8 hours
Servings: **4**

Ingredients:

- 2 pounds pork stew meat, cubed
- 1 yellow onion, sliced
- 1 cup blackberries
- ½ teaspoon rosemary, dried
- ½ teaspoon black peppercorns, crushed
- A pinch of salt and black pepper
- Juice of ½ lemon
- 2 garlic cloves, minced

Directions:

1. In your slow cooker, mix the pork with the onion, the berries and the other ingredients, toss, put the lid on and cook on Low for 8 hours.
2. Divide everything between plates and serve.

Nutritional Values (Per Serving):

Calories: 261

Carbs: 9 g
Fat: 4 g
Fiber: 8 g
Protein: 17 g

6.8 - Dill Pork Mix

Preparation time: 10 minutes
Cooking time: 45 minutes
Servings: **4**

Ingredients:

- 2 pounds pork meat, cubed
- 1 yellow onion, chopped
- 2 tablespoons olive oil
- 1 cup vegetable stock
- 1 teaspoon caraway seeds
- A pinch of salt and black pepper
- 2 tablespoons dill, chopped

Directions:

1. Heat up a pan with the oil over medium heat, add the onion and sauté for 5 minutes.
2. Add the meat and brown for 5 minutes more.
3. Add the rest of the ingredients, toss, cook over medium heat for 35 minutes, divide between plates sand serve.

Nutritional Values (Per Serving):

Calories: 300

Carbs: 12 g
Fat: 12.8 g
Fiber: 6 g
Protein: 16 g

Preparation time: 10 minutes
Cooking time: 1 hour
Servings: **4**

Ingredients:

- 2 pounds pork stew meat, cubed
- 2 tablespoons olive oil
- ½ cup vegetable stock
- 1 yellow onion, chopped
- 1 tablespoon ginger, grated
- 2 tablespoons balsamic vinegar
- A pinch of salt and black pepper
- ½ teaspoon chili powder

Directions:

1. Heat up a pan with the oil over medium heat, add the onion and the ginger and sauté for 5 minutes.
2. Add the meat and other ingredients, toss, cook over medium heat for 45 minutes more, divide between plates and serve.

Nutritional Values (Per Serving):

Calories: 280

Carbs: 12 g
Fat: 7.8 g
Fiber: 8 g
Protein: 15.6 g

Preparation time: 10 minutes
Cooking time: 30 minutes
Servings: **4**

Ingredients:

- 4 scallions, chopped
- 2 garlic cloves, minced
- 2 tablespoons olive oil
- 2 pounds pork stew meat, cubed
- 1 teaspoon sweet paprika
- A pinch of salt and black pepper
- ½ cup mustard
- 1 tablespoon chives, chopped

Directions:

1. Heat up a pan with the oil over medium heat, add the scallions and the garlic and sauté for 5 minutes.
2. Add the meat and brown it for 5 minutes.
3. Add the rest of the ingredients, toss, cook over medium heat for 20 minutes more, divide into bowls and serve.

Nutritional Values (Per Serving):

Calories: 271

Carbs: 15 g
Fat: 5 g
Fiber: 6 g
Protein: 20 g

Fish and Seafood

Preparation time: 5 minutes
Cooking time: 15 minutes
Servings: **4**

Ingredients:

- 4 salmon fillets, boneless
- 1 teaspoon chili powder
- 1 teaspoon hot paprika
- 2 tablespoons olive oil
- 2 spring onions, chopped
- A pinch of salt and black pepper
- ¼ cup fresh chives, chopped
- 1 tablespoon lemon juice

Directions:

1. Heat up a pan with the oil over medium heat, add the spring onions and sauté for 2 minutes.
2. Add the fish and cook it for 5 minutes on each side.
3. Add the rest of the ingredients, toss gently, cook for 3 minutes more, divide everything between plates and serve.

Nutritional Values (Per Serving):

Calories: 272

Carbs: 12 g
Fat: 4 g
Fiber: 2 g
Protein: 7 g

7.2 - Lemon Sea Bass

Preparation time: 5 minutes
Cooking time: 12 minutes
Servings: **4**

Ingredients:

- 4 sea bass fillets, boneless
- 2 tablespoons olive oil
- 3 spring onions, chopped
- 2 tablespoons lemon juice
- Salt and black pepper to the taste
- 2 tablespoons dill, chopped

Directions:

1. Heat up a pan with the oil over medium heat, add the onions and sauté for 2 minutes.
2. Add the fish and the other ingredients, cook everything for 5 minutes on each side, divide the mix between plates and serve.

Nutritional Values (Per Serving):

Calories: 214

Carbs: 7 g
Fat: 12 g
Fiber: 4 g
Protein: 17 g

Preparation time: 5 minutes
Cooking time: 15 minutes
Servings: **4**

Ingredients:

- 4 trout fillets, boneless
- 2 tablespoons avocado oil
- 1 cup cilantro, chopped
- 2 tablespoons lemon juice
- ½ cup coconut cream
- 1 tablespoon walnuts, chopped
- A pinch of salt and black pepper
- 3 teaspoons lemon zest, grated

Directions:

1. In a blender, combine the cilantro with the cream and the other ingredients except the fish and the oil and pulse well.
2. Heat up a pan with the oil over medium heat, add the fish and cook for 4 minutes on each side.
3. Add the cilantro sauce, toss gently and cook over medium heat for 7 minutes more.
4. Divide the mix between plates and serve.

Nutritional Values (Per Serving):

Calories: 212

Carbs: 2.9 g
Fat: 14.6 g
Fiber: 1.3 g
Protein: 18 g

Preparation time: 5 minutes
Cooking time: 20 minutes
Servings: **4**

Ingredients:

- 1 yellow onion, chopped
- 1 tablespoon olive oil
- 1 pound tuna fillets, boneless, skinless and cubed
- 1 cup tomatoes, chopped
- 1 red pepper, chopped
- 1 teaspoon sweet paprika
- 1 tablespoon coriander, chopped

Directions:

1. Heat up a pan with the oil over medium heat, add the onions and the pepper and cook for 5 minutes.
2. Add the fish and the other ingredients, cook everything for 15 minutes, divide between plates and serve.

Nutritional Values (Per Serving):

Calories: 215

Carbs: 14 g
Fat: 4 g
Fiber: 7 g
Protein: 7 g

Preparation time: 5 minutes
Cooking time: 12 minutes
Servings: **4**

Ingredients:

- 1 pound shrimp, peeled and deveined
- 2 tablespoons avocado oil
- 2 spring onions, chopped
- 2 endives, shredded
- 1 tablespoon balsamic vinegar
- 1 tablespoon chives, minced
- A pinch of sea salt and black pepper

Directions:

1. Heat up a pan with the oil over medium-high heat, add the spring onions, endives and chives, stir and cook for 4 minutes.
2. Add the shrimp and the rest of the ingredients, toss, cook over medium heat for 8 minutes more, divide into bowls and serve.

Nutritional Values (Per Serving):

Calories: 191

Fat: 3.3 g
Fiber: 8,5 Carbs: 11.3 g
Protein: 29.3 g

Preparation time: 5 minutes
Cooking time: 12 minutes
Servings: **4**

Ingredients:

- 4 tilapia fillets, boneless
- 2 tablespoons olive oil
- 2 tablespoons lemon juice
- 1 teaspoon basil, dried
- 1 tablespoon cilantro, chopped

Directions:

1. Heat up a pan with the oil over medium heat, add the fish and cook for 5 minutes on each side.
2. Add the rest of the ingredients, toss gently, cook for 2 minutes more, divide between plates and serve.

Nutritional Values (Per Serving):

Calories: 201

Carbs: 0.2 g
Fat: 8.6 g
Fiber: 0 g
Protein: 31.6 g

7.7 - Almond Scallops Mix

Preparation time: 5 minutes
Cooking time: 10 minutes
Servings: **4**

Ingredients:

- 1 pound scallops
- 2 tablespoons olive oil
- 4 scallions, chopped
- A pinch of salt and black pepper
- ½ cup mushrooms, sliced
- 2 tablespoon almonds, chopped
- 1 cup coconut cream

Directions:

1. Heat up a pan with the oil over medium heat, add the scallions and the mushrooms and sauté for 2 minutes.
2. Add the scallops and the other ingredients, toss, cook over medium heat for 8 minutes more, divide into bowls and serve.

Nutritional Values (Per Serving):

Calories: 322

Carbs: 8.1 g
Fat: 23.7 g
Fiber: 2.2 g
Protein: 21.6 g

Preparation time: 5 minutes
Cooking time: 25 minutes
Servings: **4**

Ingredients:

- 1 cup roasted red peppers, cut into strips
- 4 salmon fillets, boneless
- ¼ cup chicken stock
- 2 tablespoons olive oil
- 1 yellow onion, chopped
- 1 tablespoon cilantro, chopped
- A pinch of sea salt and black pepper

Directions:

1. Heat up a pan with the oil over medium-high heat, add the onion and sauté for 5 minutes.
2. Add the fish and cook for 5 minutes on each side.
3. Add the rest of the ingredients, introduce the pan in the oven and cook at 390 degrees F for 10 minutes.
4. Divide the mix between plates and serve.

Nutritional Values (Per Serving):

Calories: 265

Carbs: 15 g
Fat: 7 g
Fiber: 5 g
Protein: 16 g

Preparation time: 10 minutes
Cooking time: 25 minutes
Servings: **4**

Ingredients:

- 3 scallions, chopped
- 2 cups chicken stock
- 1 pound cod fillets, boneless and cubed
- 1 cup black quinoa
- 2 tablespoons olive oil
- 2 celery stalks, chopped
- A pinch of salt and black pepper
- 1 tablespoon coriander, chopped

Directions:

1. Heat up a pan with the oil over medium-high heat, add the scallions and the celery and sauté for 5 minutes.
2. Add the fish and cook for 5 minutes more.
3. Add the rest of the ingredients, toss, cook over medium heat for 15 minutes more, divide everything between plates and serve.

Nutritional Values (Per Serving):

Calories: 261

Carbs: 14 g
Fat: 4 g
Fiber: 6 g
Protein: 7 g

7.10 - Cinnamon Scallops

Preparation time: 10 minutes
Cooking time: 20 minutes
Servings: **4**

Ingredients:

- 2 tablespoons olive oil
- 2 jalapenos, chopped
- 1 pound sea scallops
- A pinch of salt and black pepper
- ¼ teaspoon cinnamon powder
- 1 teaspoon garam masala
- 1 teaspoon coriander, ground
- 1 teaspoon cumin, ground
- 2 tablespoons cilantro, chopped

Directions:

1. Heat up a pan with the oil over medium heat, add the jalapenos, cinnamon and the other ingredients except the scallops and cook for 10 minutes.
2. Add the rest of the ingredients, toss, cook for 10 minutes more, divide into bowls and serve.

Nutritional Values (Per Serving):

Calories: 251

Carbs: 11 g
Fat: 4 g
Fiber: 4 g
Protein: 17 g

Desserts

Preparation time: 5 minutes
Cooking time: 0 minutes
Servings: **4**

Ingredients:

- 1 cup blackberries
- 1 cup pineapple, peeled and cubed
- 1 tablespoon coconut oil, melted
- ¾ cup coconut cream
- 2 tablespoons maple syrup

Directions:

1. In your blender, combine the berries with the pineapple and the other ingredients, pulse well, divide into bowls and serve cold.

Nutritional Values (Per Serving):

Calories: 120

Carbs: 6 g
Fat: 3 g
Fiber: 3 g
Protein: 8 g

Preparation time: 10 minutes
Cooking time: 0 minutes
Servings: **2**

Ingredients:

- 2 cups mango, peeled and c hopped
- 1 cup orange juice
- 1 tablespoon ginger, grated
- 1 teaspoon turmeric powder

Directions:

1. In your blender, combine the mango with the juice and the other ingredients, pulse well, divide into 2 glasses and serve cold.

Nutritional Values (Per Serving):

Calories: 100

Carbs: 4 g
Fat: 1 g
Fiber: 2 g
Protein: 5 g

Preparation time: 10 minutes
Cooking time: 0 minutes
Servings: **4**

Ingredients:

- 1 avocado, peeled, pitted and chopped
- 1 big banana, peeled and chopped
- 1 mango, peeled and cubed
- 1 tablespoon honey
- ½ cup grapes, halved
- 1 tablespoon lime juice
- 2 teaspoons lime zest, grated

Directions:

1. In a bowl, combine the avocado with the banana and the other ingredients, toss, divide into small bowls and serve.

Nutritional Values (Per Serving):

Calories: 207

Carbs: 31.1 g
Fat: 10.3 g
Fiber: 5.8 g
Protein: 2.1 g

Preparation time: 10 minutes
Cooking time: 15 minutes
Servings: **4**

Ingredients:

- 2 tablespoons lime juice
- 2 cups watermelon, peeled and cubed
- 1 tablespoon chicory root powder
- 2 tablespoons flax meal mixed with 4 tablespoons water

Directions:

---

1. In a small pot, combine the watermelon with the other ingredients, toss, simmer over medium heat for 15 minutes, divide into bowls and serve cold.

Nutritional Values (Per Serving):

Calories: 161

Carbs: 8 g
Fat: 4 g
Fiber: 2 g
Protein: 5 g

Preparation time: 2 hours
Cooking time: 0 minutes
Servings: **4**

Ingredients:

- 1/3 cup natural coconut butter, melted
- 1 and ½ tablespoons coconut oil
- 2 tablespoons orange juice
- ½ teaspoon orange zest, grated
- 1 tablespoons honey

Directions:

1. In a bowl, combine the coconut butter with the oil and the other ingredients, stir well, scoop into a square pan, spread well, cut into bars, keep in the freezer for 2 hours and serve.

Nutritional Values (Per Serving):

Calories: 72

Carbs: 8 g
Fat: 4 g
Fiber: 2 g
Protein: 6 g

8.6 - Coconut Apple Bars

Preparation time: 10 minutes
Cooking time: 25 minutes
Servings: **6**

Ingredients:

- ½ cup coconut cream
- 1 cup apples, peeled, cored and chopped
- ½ cup maple syrup
- 1 teaspoon vanilla extract
- ½ cup almond flour
- 2 eggs, whisked
- 1 teaspoon baking powder

Directions:

1. In a blender, combine the cream with the apples and the other ingredients and pulse well.
2. Pour this into a baking dish lined with parchment paper, bake in the oven at 370 degrees F for 25 minutes, cool down, cut into bars and serve.

Nutritional Values (Per Serving):

Calories: 200

Carbs: 12 g
Fat: 3 g
Fiber: 4 g
Protein: 11 g

Preparation time: 10 minutes
Cooking time: 0 minutes
Servings: **4**

Ingredients:

- 2 teaspoons lime juice
- 1 pound pears, cored, peeled and chopped
- 1 pound strawberries, chopped
- 1 cup coconut cream

Directions:

1. In a blender, combine the pears with strawberries and the other ingredients, pulse well, divide into bowls and serve.

Nutritional Values (Per Serving):

Calories: 100

Carbs: 8 g
Fat: 2 g
Fiber: 3 g
Protein: 5 g

Preparation time: 10 minutes
Cooking time: 30 minutes
Servings: **6**

Ingredients:

- 2 pears, cored, peeled and chopped
- 2 cups coconut flour
- 1 cup dates, pitted
- 2 eggs, whisked
- 1 teaspoon vanilla extract
- 1 teaspoon baking soda
- ½ cup coconut oil, melted
- ½ teaspoon cinnamon powder

Directions:

1. In a bowl, combine the pears with the flour and the other ingredients, whisk well, pour into a cake pan and bake at 360 degrees F for 30 minutes.
2. Cool down, slice and serve.

Nutritional Values (Per Serving):

Calories: 160

Carbs: 8 g
Fat: 7 g
Fiber: 4 g
Protein: 4. g

Preparation time: 2 hours
Cooking time: 0 minutes
Servings: **4**

Ingredients:

- 2 cups coconut cream
- 1 watermelon, peeled and chopped
- 2 avocados, peeled, pitted and chopped
- 1 tablespoon honey
- 2 teaspoons lemon juice

Directions:

1. In a blender, combine the watermelon with the cream and the other ingredients, pulse well, divide into bowls and keep in the fridge for 2 hours before serving.

Nutritional Values (Per Serving):

Calories: 121

Carbs: 6 g
Fat: 2 g
Fiber: 2 g
Protein: 5 g

Preparation time: 10 minutes
Cooking time: 0 minutes
Servings: **4**

Ingredients:

- ½ cup dates, pitted
- ½ teaspoon vanilla extract
- 1 cup almonds, chopped
- 1 cup blackberries
- 1 tablespoon maple syrup
- 1 tablespoon coconut oil, melted

Directions:

1. In a bowl, combine the berries with the almonds and the other ingredients, toss, divide into small cups and serve.

Nutritional Values (Per Serving):

Calories: 130

Carbs: 12 g
Fat: 5 g
Fiber: 5 g
Protein: 4 g

Conclusion

Autoimmune responses to some diseases, infections or injuries lead to inflammation. This book tackles the importance of inflammation and how it can be managed with an anti-inflammatory diet. It discusses issues like what foods help reduce inflammation, lifestyle changes to keep inflammation at bay, and some common sources of inflammation that also need special attention.

Inflammation is a healthy process of our body. It protects us from diseases and makes sure that the cells do not get hurt. The immune system is what makes this happen, but when it becomes chronic, then it becomes an inflammatory disease that will cause trouble.

This disease will lead to different problems and can even attack our most important organs. The best thing to do is prevent it from happening in the first place.

In the second place it's important to find the signs of chronic inflammation early so you can limit and reverse the impact it is having on your health. Chronic inflammation is a root cause for many long-term diseases, so ignoring these signs can cause major problems in your health.

If you have the inflammatory disease, then you need to take care of it. The goal is to make sure that you don't get out of control and then have to do medical interventions. We want you to prevent yourself from getting too bad.

For those suffering from inflammation, this cookbook is a godsend. It answers almost all questions that you could have as well as giving guidance about how to contact your doctor for the rest of your concerns.

One way that has been shown to be effective against the condition is adopting an anti-inflammatory diet.

Lucky for us, many lifestyle changes can be performed to stop and reverse this disease process when it is still in its advanced stages, should we choose not to halt progression by taking medication.

Adopting an anti-inflammatory diet plan is one major change you can make in your lifestyle. It features healthy, nutritious and satisfying dishes without a significant compromise on flavor - unlike the weight-loss diets which often leave people very hungry.

We have proved the myth of a healthy diet being tasteless wrong by publishing the previous recipes from all over the world.

Adding food items with anti-inflammatory benefits to your diet, one of the most common and beneficial methods for fighting inflammation, is highly regarded.

A recent study found that anti-inflammatory food eaten with a healthy lifestyle has proven to be much more effective than medicines. And it's not only for those who have regular exercise but also for athletes, like professional football players, where surgery is often necessary because of wear and tear on their body cells.

This anti-inflammatory diet book includes recipes that will help alleviate your pain and treatments that other books have not tackled. It has everything you need to know about inflammation, whether it is dietary, or a chronic illness.

We hope that the information you read in this book gives you a better understanding of how immune dysfunction results from chronic inflammation, and empower you to take control of your own diet plan so it supports your body's innate healing abilities.

Our recipes are just the beginning. Use them as a guide to create many of your dishes that follow the diet plan. Just make sure you consider the proper ingredients and food groups when preparing meals. And for maximum effects, please be aware of our Anti-Inflammatory Diet food guide

Now that you have learnt about the benefits of a anti-inflammatory diet, it is time to take action. Identify signs and symptoms of chronic inflammation and make safe lifestyle changes to prevent further health complications.

Logistically, implementing the anti-inflammatory diet may be a challenge in the beginning as you establish new habits and regime. However, once you are able to adjust your scheduled for regular portions of food, it will become an ingrained part of your routine.

A diet with anti-inflammatory foods can have many positive effects, such as improved energy, better mental function, a stronger immune system and less chronic pain. Additionally, it could lead to healthier weight loss or overall better health outcomes.

If you have been ready to experience these changes, don't wait any longer and start putting your knowledge from this book into action.

With so much information available online and offline, it becomes very easy for the reader to get confused or lose interest. This adds to the pain that inflammation has caused already. With this book's help, you'll have all of your questions answered, no need to worry about anything.

Beat the pain while you enjoy these foods!

Thank you for reading this book. It is my hope that it provided you with valuable information and the tools to accomplish your goals, whatever they may be.

Indexes in Alphabetical Order

Index of Recipes

W

Index of Ingredients

CPSIA information can be obtained
at www.ICGtesting.com
Printed in the USA
BVHW041721090621
609091BV00016B/2530

9 781803 113913